How to Give a Home Manicure & Pedicure

Copyright © 2013

Printed by: CreateSpace, Amazon. Com Company (2014)
Available on Kindle and other devices.
All rights reserved. No part of this publication may be copied, reproduced in any format, by any means, electronic or otherwise, without prior consent from the copyright owner and publisher of this book

How to Give a Home Manicure & Pedicure

By: A.E Wilson

Table of Contents

Manicure---- 4

Pedicure-----6

Chapter 1 - Benefits of Getting a Manicure---8

Chapter 2 - A Day of Pampering---10

Chapter 3 - The First Step- The Hand Soak---14

Chapter 4 - Trimming and Shaping the Fingernails---17

Chapter 5 - The Hand Massage---20

Chapter 6 - Building an Iconic Nail Polish Collection---23

Chapter 7 - Applying Nail Polish and Simple Nail Art---26

Chapter 8 - Giving Your Loved One a Special Manicure Treat- The Gel Manicure---29

Chapter 9 - Hand Care and Manicure Maintenance---32

Chapter 10-Benefits of Getting a Pedicure---34

Chapter 11 - Who Should and Shouldn't Get a Pedicure?---37

Chapter 12 - Setting the Stage for a Pedicure Party---40

Chapter 13 - Items You'll Need to Prepare for a Pedicure---44

Chapter 14 - The First Step- A Foot Soak----47

Chapter 15 - Cutting and Shaping the Toenails---49

Chapter 16- Exfoliation---51

Chapter 17 – Massage---53

Chapter 18 - The Final Touches- Buffing and Polishing-56

Manicure

In today's fast-paced lifestyle, we often forget to give time to the people who matter most- our family and friends. Sure, grabbing a quick bite to eat or a day out in the mall with them is fun, but if you want a unique bonding experience that will allow you to catch up and pamper them at the same time, then giving them a manicure is the best way to do this.

Ever wanted to learn how to give a professional-grade manicure right in the comforts of your own home? Do you want to treat your family and friends to one right now? This book will give you a step-by-step guide on doing a great manicure that your loved ones will surely appreciate!

Know the reasons why it's good to get a manicure. Learn the health benefits of getting one, and how a manicure can be part of one's personal style. Nowadays, it's not just paint on the nails, it's an accessory too.

Find out how to give a one on one manicure session, or turn it into an afternoon of pampering. Chapter 2 shows you how to organize a manicure party for any occasion, whether it's going to be the theme for a gathering of girlfriends, a treat for elderly relatives, a kiddie party for your very girly daughter or niece, or a bridal shower for your best friend.

Learn how to make a hand soak a relaxing and therapeutic part of a manicure, and the different things that you can add to it to make it more special.

Chapter 4 gives you a guide on trimming and shaping the nails which is the most crucial aspect to any well-executed manicure. Learn how to do this safely and neatly. You'll be amazed how easy it is.

One of the most pleasant parts of the manicure is the hand massage, which is covered in chapter 5. Discover how to give a relaxing and soothing massage, and find out what are the best hand creams are out there in the market today.

If you are in the habit of collecting the "it" colors of nail polish, why not build an iconic nail polish collection? Chapter 6 tells all about the nail polish brands and shades that have sparked world-wide trends and have been found featured in certain films and gracing the fingertips of well-known celebrities and tastemakers. Your family and friends will be entertained by the stories behind the names of famous nail polishes, not to mention the great things they'll say once they see the way these colors look on their own nails.

Learn how to apply nail polish the classic way and add a fun spin to it with some simple nail art. Also, find out how easy it is to give a gel manicure at home. With the right products, you can do a salon-worthy manicure that's sure to last for a long time.

Know the importance of hand and nail care and the tips and advice you can give to your loved ones to take care of their hands and nails, and how to maintain the manicure until it's time to have it redone.

All these you can get from this book. So read on and find out how easy and fulfilling it is to give a manicure to your family and friends!

Pedicure

There are a lot of ways to show your family and friends that you care for them and appreciate them. You can cook them a special meal, take them out for lunch or a cup of coffee, or give them tickets to a show or sports event that they would really love. But what if you happen to be short on cash? There's another way to show that you care- and that is by giving them a pedicure!

If you're hesitant about giving a pedicure, fear not. This book will give you a step by step guide on doing a professional grade pedicure that your loved ones will truly appreciate. You'll be amazed at how easy it is to do yourself.

Learn about the benefits of having a pedicure and how it can be an instant mood lifter. And did you know that pedicures have health benefits too? Aside from having pretty, painted toenails, a pedicure can even alleviate certain foot aches and pains.
Know who should and shouldn't get a pedicure. Not all people are advised to have one, so it pays to be informed right before you pick up that brand new bottle of nail polish.

For an added dose of fun, why not turn a pedicure session into a pedicure party? In Chapter 3 you will get a lot of helpful tips on how to organize one. From fixing up the party area, to getting ideas for yummy snacks to serve and fun giveaways for all your guests, it's all here for you.

Discover the things that you should have on hand to perform a pedicure. Chapter 4 will give you a list of the basic tools and other things that you'll need.

Find out why a foot bath is the first step to every great pedicure, and the things that you can add to it to make it an even more pleasant and soothing experience for your loved ones.

Well-trimmed and neatly shaped nails are the foundation of a good pedicure. Learn how to cut and shape nails safely in chapter 6.

The next chapter tells all about exfoliation and gives you the best- and cheapest- exfoliant that is perfect for a pedicure. And the best thing about it is you can make it in your own kitchen!

Know how to give a relaxing foot and leg massage, which is definitely one of the most pleasant parts of a pedicure.

Finally, learn the proper way to apply nail polish for a professional finish. Plus, know the top 5 nail polish shades that have withstood the test of time.

This book shows you that pedicures can be nurturing, caring, and fun for your family, friends, and you! So read on and let's get started on learning how to pamper the people who matter the most.

Chapter 1 - Benefits of Getting a Manicure

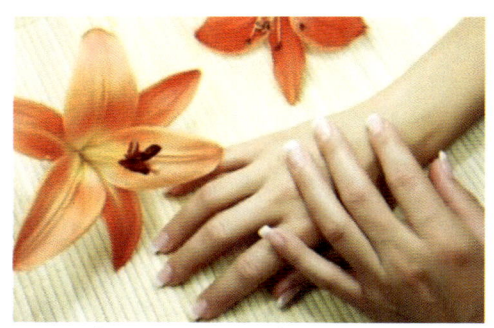

It's true that you only get one chance to make a good first impression. The way we present ourselves says a lot about the kind of person we are. It's a well known fact that people gravitate towards those who look neat, clean, and well groomed. And there's nothing like clean, well-manicured hands to say that a person is put together.

Nowadays, it's not just women who tend to get manicures. Men are in on the action too, specially businessmen and executives who want their hands to look clean. In New York, there is a continuing proliferation of nail salons which seem to sprout up in every corner, offering manicures for about $15. Because there is such an emphasis on good grooming in this city, these nail salons are making a tidy profit from all their customers from all walks of life.

Even those who live far away from the hustle and bustle of the city will surely appreciate a manicure. For instance, those who are nearest and dearest to us- our family and friends- would surely love the benefits that accompany a good manicure.

A manicure can be a source of relaxation. It allows people to stop what they're doing and inject a little pampering time in their busy schedules. It's an excellent way to treat a friend, especially if they are in need of a little TLC.
Aside from relaxation, a manicure can also help a person stay healthy. Clean hands and fingernails are essential to health, and regularly taking the time to remove deep seated dirt from underneath the nails is a good practice to avoid sickness.

Hands are also lavished with much attention during a manicure. A massage done with hydrating moisturizers and creams will surely help dry nails and cuticles, and will also increase blood circulation, making hands look younger and feel supple. Also, aching joints and wrists will be relieved of pain, probably brought about by daily chores or by daily tapping away at the computer keyboard.

This is also an inexpensive way to accessorize and spice up an outfit. With nail polish being available in every color and hue imaginable, and nail art designs that take inspiration from everything around us, a manicure is surely a more affordable way to give a woman's style a little pizzazz. It can help a person express her personality, because the nail colors and designs that she will choose are an extension of her personal style.

For you, the giver of the manicure, this can be a good way to bond with your loved ones and show them that you care for their well-being. It is a generous, selfless act that enables you to spend a little time and effort for the ones you love. All you have to do is to set the time to do it and have the materials and other equipment on hand. It is also important for you to be relaxed and in a positive mindset to give the manicure, so that you and loved ones will enjoy every minute of it.

Chapter 2 - A Day of Pampering

A one on one manicure can be soothing and relaxing. But to make this even better, why not organize a manicure party? This theme is versatile and can work for any situation or age group. Get a bunch of girlfriends to hang out at your place and it's an instant gabfest, just another reason to get together, get pampered and catch up. Invite your elderly relatives and let them reminisce about the good old days while you shower them with attention and paint their nails. Stumped about what to do for your daughter's birthday party? Turn it into a spa party and invite her best friends for a fun and delightful day for everyone. Got to throw a bridal shower for your sister? Make it a spa party!

To make any event successful, take the time to plan ahead and organize. Give yourself a week to prepare and send out the invitations. Plan on having it down to 1 is to 3 when it comes to the number of manicure givers to recipients. For a simple get together with your friends, this is the perfect ratio for it, so invite no more than 3 at a time for an afternoon of pampering. For your elderly relatives, the same number of guests is also recommended. For a little girl's birthday party, there will probably be more than 3 kids awaiting a manicure so it's a good idea to have extra manicurists on hand (call the other moms and see if they'd like to pitch in). The same goes for a spa-themed bridal shower.

Here are a few tips to do the following manicure-related events:

The Girlfriend Get-Together

Along with 2 or 3 of your closest friends or siblings, you can have this easily at your very own living room. Simply provide comfortable chairs and some throw pillows for plushy comfort. Play a few episodes of HBOs Girls or Game of Thrones or even the first season of Sex and the City or Friends on the DVD player. Serve food before giving manicures. Light fare such as sandwiches with the crusts cut off and tea are ideal and easy to make and serve. Send your guests home with a new bottle of nail polish as a party favor.

It's All in the Family

Your aunts and other relatives, specially the elderly ones will surely appreciate that you took the time to care for them. Prepare your living room the same way, with comfortable seating. This time, show some classics on your TV screen. Movies starring Audrey Hepburn or Marilyn Monroe, or MGM musicals will be enjoyed and applauded. Serve some coffee cake, sandwiches and coffee and tea. Give each loved one a pocket-sized bottle of hand lotion as a token.

Kids Just Wanna Have Fun

For a kids' party it might be good to have some extra hands to deal with all the little girls wanting a manicure. Have your daughter invite no more than 9 of her friends. For every 3 girls, plan on having one person to do their manicure. It might be a great idea to call some of the other moms and ask if they would like to participate. Once you have your manicure team, you can get them to wear pink shirts, or aprons with "The Spa Squad" written on them. And yes, you should wear the same thing too! Decorate your living room or patio with lots of pink or girly paraphernalia. Hello Kitty or Barbie-themed items are specially loved by little fashionistas. Add some movie posters of kid-friendly flicks and set the DVD to play the same kind of movies. Harry Potter or the High School Musical movies are great choices. Or show some animated films such as Tangled, Brave, or Epic. Disney and Pixar have a lot of movies to choose from, so take your pick. Serve kid-friendly fare before the manicures such as mini grilled cheese sandwiches and fruit juice to keep the hunger pangs away. Serve more food after the manicures are done so your child's guests can partake of typical party food such as birthday cake. Before they leave, treat your little guests to some mini bottles of sparkly nail polish.

Bridal Shower Extraordinaire

If you have a sister or a friend who would like to celebrate minus the ruckus and noise of a typical rowdy bridal shower, a spa-themed get-together will be more appropriate perhaps for this time. Make it special and send out invitations. Again, be mindful of the manicurist to recipient ratio. You can do this at a hotel room and have about 12 of the bride's closest relatives and friends to come over. Have them bring 2 bottles of nail polish each so you'll have a wide selection of colors to choose from. Have some light but filling snacks sent up such as quiche and canapés. Send your guests home with Essie Nail Polish in Ballet Slipper, a favorite of brides everywhere and a true classic.

These are just some ideas to organize a manicure party. So invite a few people, have the music, movies and food ready, and let the good times roll!

Chapter 3 - The First Step- The Hand Soak

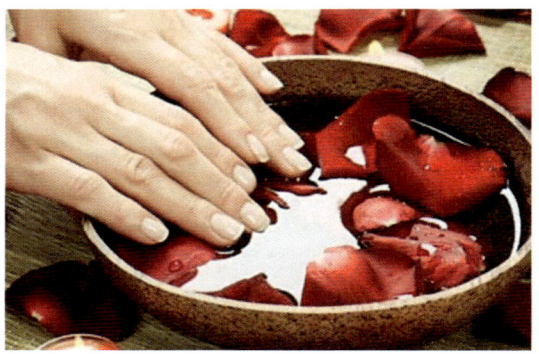

Whenever we watch a nail salon scene in a movie, chances are there's always somebody soaking their fingertips in a bowlful of scented water. This however, is not just for cinematic purposes. A hand soak is vital before starting a manicure. It removes dirt, softens the nails and cuticles to prepare them for trimming, and disinfects the whole hand. Along with the hand soak, most professional salons also do a "hand spa", which is a fancy way to refer to the exfoliation process that follows the soak.

To begin, prepare the following items:
- A small plastic basin
- Warm water
- Non drying liquid hand soap
- A few drops of essential oil
- A body or face scrub, try St. Ives Apricot Scrub for a clean yet moisturized feel
- A soft and clean hand towel

Start by having your loved one take off any jewelry such as rings, bracelets or watches. Prepare the hand soak by pouring in some warm water into the basin, then add a few squirts of liquid hand soap. If skin is suffering from dryness, some moisturizing hand soap would be ideal such as Dove liquid soap.
Create a few suds in the water, then add a few drops of essential oil.

There are different types of oils in the market that your family and friends will love. Here are some recommendations:

To relieve stress

Lavender oil has a calming and relaxing effect, very effective to reduce stress. It is also used in some baby products to help promote a good night's sleep. However, if used excessively this type of essential oil can keep you awake and "wired" so, limit the use to about 3 to 4 drops only in the hand soak.

To refresh tired hands

Peppermint or eucalyptus essential oils are ideal to refresh the hands. The sharp, minty aroma decreases fatigue and can also help clear a stuffy nose.

For a soft, feminine scent

Rose oil is widely preferred by those who like softly scented hands. This is also good for people who are suffering from depression because the scent is known to help uplift and comfort.

For a quick hit of sugary sweetness

Vanilla oil is comforting and smells like home, since it reminds people of the smells that emanates from their mother's kitchen. Nowadays, vanilla is often blended into perfumes and colognes and it has a sweet and creamy, almost edible smell.

Let your loved ones soak their hands in for about 5 minutes, then one hand at a time, apply an exfoliating scrub to their hands and forearms with an upwards scrubbing motion. This removes deep seated dirt and reveals softer, smoother and more even-toned skin. Regular exfoliation of the hands and arms also encourages faster skin cell turnover, so skin looks better immediately. After scrubbing, rinse with some more warm water, and pat hands and arms with a soft towel.

Now that the first step is done, you're ready to move on to trimming and shaping the nails, which will be discussed in the next chapter.

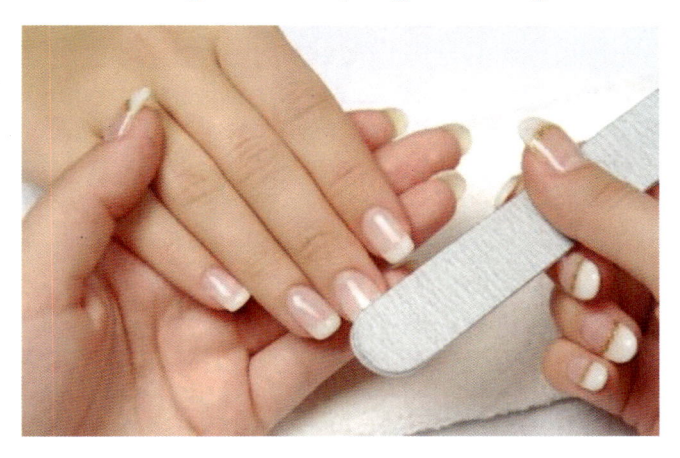

Chapter 4 - Trimming and Shaping the Fingernails

This is probably the most important part of a manicure, yes, even more so than polishing the nails. It is a known fact that neatly trimmed and shaped nails says a lot about a person. This should be done with much care to avoid nicking the recipient of the manicure.

During the early 80's, long fingernails were all the rage and some women even used acrylic nails to add length to their fingertips. Nowadays, shorter styles are more popular. Although celebrities like Rihanna, Adele and Beyonce sport long, pointed nails, many prefer short, rounded nails for their versatility and practicality.

Before trimming the nails, ask your loved ones how short they want their nails to be. Ideally, the length of the nail should extend slightly above the fingertip. However, if they want their nails a little longer than that, then it would do to oblige. However, if your friend's nails are brittle and prone to breakage, shorter nails would look best and are more low maintenance.

How to Give a Home
Manicure & Pedicure

First, get your things ready: a nail clipper, emery boards, orange sticks, cuticle remover, cuticle nippers or scissors. The cuticle nippers or scissors should be sterilized, and provide each person you'll give a manicure to their own emery board and orange stick to avoid cross contamination.

The best time to trim the nails is while they are still soft from the hand soak. Trim the nails, starting from one side going to the other. Snip carefully, and avoid starting the cut from the middle of the nail since this can cause tiny cracks at the top of the nail. Make sure that all the nails are of the same length.

File the nails with quick, side to side short strokes. The best way to do this is with an emery board, and not a metal file as this can be damaging to the nails. Don't skip this step because filing refines the shape of the nail.

Now it's time to push back the cuticles, which is an essential step when doing a manicure. Use a few drops of cuticle remover on each nail to soften the cuticles, making them easier to push back with an orange stick. Using the flat end (not the pointy end), gently push back the cuticle towards the base of the nail. Then, run the pointy end lightly along the base to dislodge any dry skin. It's best not to cut the cuticles because they protect the nails against infection and bacteria. Use the nippers or manicure scissors to carefully trim any hangnails.

All the materials that were mentioned in this chapter should be carefully sterilized between each use, particularly the nail clippers, manicure scissors and nippers. To do this, salons use an autoclave, a devise that sterilizes manicure equipment using heat. At home, you can disinfect your tools by saturating a cotton swab with 70 percent isopropyl alcohol, then using that to clean the cutting edges of your tools. Keep all your manicure equipment in a box or any container that has a lid on it. Some people like to repurpose an inexpensive tool box or cosmetic caddy for their nail implements. In a pinch, even those disposable, microwavable plastic containers will do. Also, keep your tools away from dust and moisture.

Chapter 5 - The Hand Massage

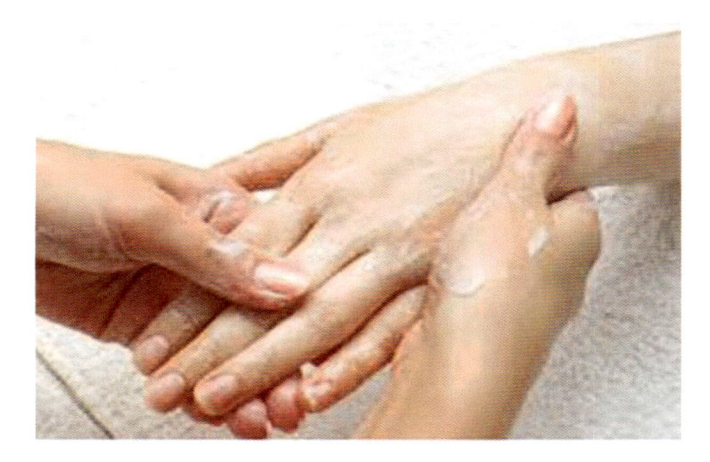

A hand massage is one of the most heavenly and relaxing things that one could get. Aside from a manicure, it's also one of the best free gifts that you can give a loved one. Our hands do a lot of work from the moment we wake up until the time that we go to sleep. So if the recipient is a stay at home mom, she's probably worn out from doing chores and errands. If your loved one works at an office, chances are her hands are probably in need of a break from tapping out on the computer keyboard. An elderly relative might be suffering from lack of attention and touch, which causes loneliness. This can be remedied by a hand massage, which is a form of touch therapy to help maintain physical and emotional wellness. No matter who receives a hand massage, your efforts will surely be appreciated.

Before you start, remember that a massage has to be soothing and not painful. It might help to ask your loved one if the pressure you're applying is just right, so you can ease up whenever needed. Also, make sure that you spend an equal length of time working on both hands. More importantly, do not give a massage to people who have circulatory problems or arthritis.

The massage should be done prior to applying the nail polish to avoid smudging or smearing the polish. You should have the following things on hand:

- Hand cream- creams specially formulated for the hands are richer and thicker than ordinary lotions. Some good creams are The Body Shop Wild Rose Hand Cream, Avon Moisture Therapy Intensive Hand Cream, Eucerin Intensive Repair Extra Enriched Hand Crème, and L'Occitane Shea Butter Hand Cream.

- A soft hand towel

Make sure that your hands are warm and relaxed before you massage your relative or friend. To begin, start with the person's dominant hand and apply a small amount of hand cream. Rub the top of the hand gently, then turn it over and work on the palm. Gently apply pressure around the palm in a circular motion.

With your thumb on the palm and the rest of your fingers gripping the back of the hand, apply steady pressure starting at the base of the little finger, going towards the wrist. Repeat for all fingers.

Next do some finger pulls, starting with the littlest finger, grasp the finger from the base, and pull towards the tip slowly. Don't use a fast, jerky motion because this might dislocate the finger.

Then, work on the palm by using your thumb to apply steady pressure in a circular motion, starting from the base of the thumb in a clockwise motion.

End the massage by holding the wrist and shaking it gently to relieve any stiffness. Do the same thing to the other hand.

Wipe away any extra hand cream as this can prevent the nail polish from adhering to the nails. Use a soft, clean towel to do this.

Now, it's time to do the fun part- applying nail polish, which will be discussed in the next chapter.

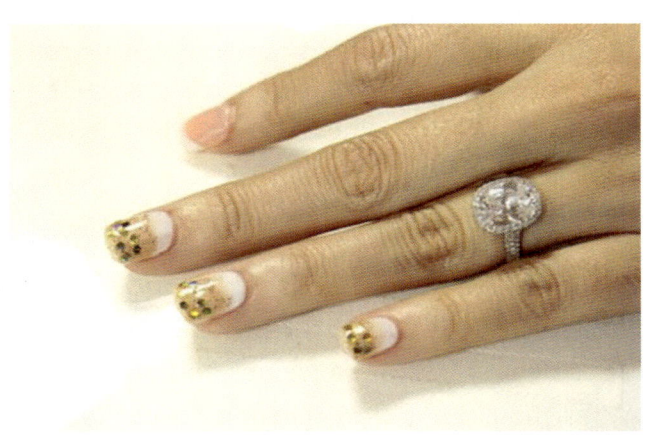

Chapter 6 - Building an Iconic Nail Polish Collection

The most fun part of a manicure is polishing the nails with vibrant colors and attempting to do designs more commonly known as nail art. With all the nail polish brands available in the market, this is a quick, easy and affordable way to spice up one's style. It's also very easy to change your look just with a quick swipe of polish remover and a fresh coat of lacquer.

Nail polish trends have also been evident throughout the decades as we witnessed the evolution of the "it" colors of the season. Case in point, in 1994, Chanel came out with a deep red and black nail polish which was created to mimic the color of dried blood, aptly named Vamp. It immediately became a hit and just flew out of stores which carried the nail polish. It also helped that Uma Thurman wore the color in Pulp Fiction during that iconic dance scene with John Travolta. After that, other brands came up with their own version of the black-red nail color, but most women who jumped on the Vamp craze can attest that nothing compares to it.

If you're on a quest to build a wardrobe of iconic nail colors, here is a list of nail polish colors and brands that have made an impact throughout the years, and will surely bring a smile to your loved ones' faces as you regale them with the story behind each bottle while painting their nails.

- **OPI I'm Not Really a Waitress**
  - This is a classic red nail polish that works on everyone. This shimmery red nail polish has often made the cut in every Best of Beauty List in magazines and blogs for over 10 years now, as the color is truly flattering on anyone, regardless of the skin tone. Susan Weiss-Finchmann, the creator of OPI nail polishes also said that this polish was named as such because it was inspired by wanna be actresses in Hollywood who waited tables while waiting for a callback on their audition. They would often say "I'm not really a waitress…" Hence, the cute and memorable name for this gorgeous red nail polish.

- **Essie Ballet Slippers**
  - A classic light pink with a sheer finish, this nail polish is a favorite of brides and fashion stylists for its versatility and clean effect on the hands. It's the quintessential "rich lady" shade of polish and it was even mentioned in the best-selling novel The Devil Wears Prada. It is also favored by lifestyle gurus and TV chefs such as Martha Stewart, Giada de Laurentiis and Ina Garten.

- **Nars Schiap**

    A vibrant, shocking pink, this nail polish is named after Elsa Schiaparelli, an Italian fashion designer who's widely known as Coco Chanel's greatest rival. This shade of pink was often used by the designer and soon she became associated with the color. Though the shade looks intimidating in the bottle, it surprisingly has a very flattering effect on hands, specially on short nails.

Add to this collection a bottle of Chanel Vamp, and viola! You've got your very own iconic collection of nail polish which you can use to give a professional manicure to your loved ones.

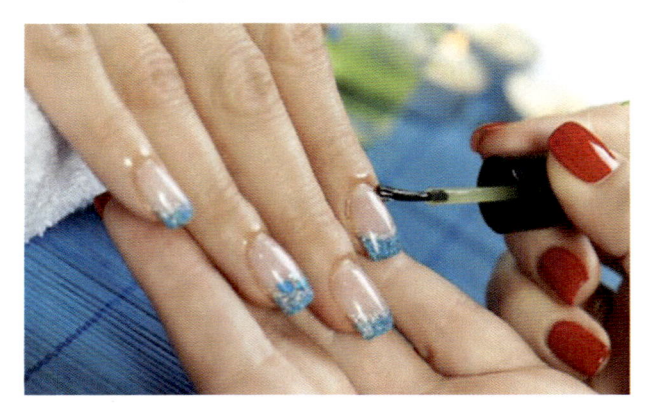

Chapter 7 - Applying Nail Polish and Simple Nail Art

Now we've come to the final part of the manicure- applying nail polish. When done properly, it can last for about one week without chipping. Proper application also ensures a glassy, smooth finish.

Before brushing on nail polish, make sure that your friend's nails are completely free of lotion or cream, so go over all 10 digits with a cotton ball soaked with polish remover. Make sure that no trace of lint from the cotton stays on the nails as this can flub the manicure.

Prepare the following items:
- Basecoat- this is the first layer of the manicure. A basecoat protects the nail from stains and discoloration. Good ones to try are Sally Hansen base coat, Zoya, and Orly's Bonder.

- Nail polish- preferably fresh bottles of nail polish. If the formula starts to separate in the bottle, it's time to get new nail polish. Old ones tend to be gloppy and that makes it more difficult to paint on a nice, even finish.

- Top coat- the final layer of the manicure. This gives nails a glossy shine. Try Seche Vite Dry Fast Top Coat to cut down on drying time.

- Orange stick, cotton and polish remover

Start by applying one coat of basecoat. Apply it in 3 strokes- down the middle of the nail, then once on either side of it. Make sure to paint from the base of the cuticle, going towards the tip of the nail.

Once the base coat is in place, grab a bottle of nail polish and roll it between your hands to make it easier to brush on. Then, swipe the brush against the inside opening of the bottle. You'll find that this move will leave just the right amount of nail polish for one thin coat. Go over the nail using the 3-stroke method again. Once you've painted all 10 nails, go over them once again with a second coat of nail polish. This will bring out the true color and luster of the nail polish. Finish with one thin layer of topcoat.

There will be some polish that might go beyond the cuticle border, so take an orange stick, wrap a bit of cotton around it, dip it in nail polish remover and go over the base of the cuticle slowly with it. Do the same on both sides of the nail to remove excess polish. Do this for all 10 digits, and now you're done!

If you're feeling particularly artsy, now would be a good time to do some simple nail art using nail polish pens. Sally Hansen and Migi Nail Art both have a wide selection of colors, and because they're in pen form, it's easier to draw designs on the nails. To start, you can attempt to do the simplest thing first- a French manicure. After painting the whole nail a pale pink color such as Essie Ballet Slippers, take a white nail art pen and go over the tip of the nail with it, drawing all through the arc of the nail tip. Top it off with a thin layer of topcoat.

If you'd like to give your loved one a special treat, you can give her a gel manicure. Read on through the next chapter to find out how easy it is to do at home.

Chapter 8 - Giving Your Loved One a Special Manicure Treat- The Gel Manicure

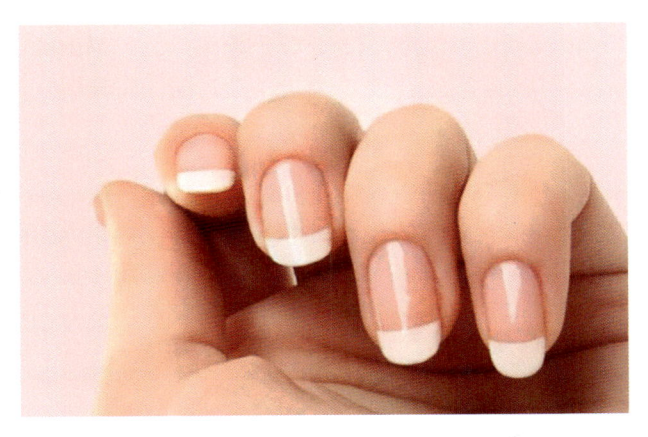

Gel manicures are a special treat that you can give your loved ones if you want them to have a manicure that lasts for a really long time. We're talking about 2 weeks here, with no chips. And the manicure dries in about 1 minute, so there's no need to sit around and wait for about 30 minutes for nails to dry completely. Sounds great, right?

How is that possible? Well, think of regular nail polish as paint, and gel manicures as plastic. It dries in a different way and it requires a moisture-free surface so it can adhere well. For this reason, you will have to perform a dry manicure, meaning, you have to skip the hand soak. Cuticles have to be groomed without using water, and nails have to be wiped down with an alcohol based cleanser to remove any oily residue. Then, each layer of polish has to be cured using an LED lamp. If this sounds complicated, don't worry. The good news is, there are a lot of at-home gel manicure kits that are in the market, and it's easier to do than you think.

Several brands that stand out are Mally Beauty 24/7 Professional Gel Nail Polish System, Orly Smartgels Starter Kit, Gelish Mini Basix Kit and Sephora by OPI Gelshine Gel Manicure System. Budget-wise, the Gelish kit is the most affordable at only $50, followed by Orly at $60.

To start, protect the surface that you'll be working on by covering it with an old table cloth or an old towel, basically something that you wouldn't mind getting stained. Then, lay out everything from the kit. A basic kit will include a small UV or LED lamp, a nail cleanser, a base coat, one colored polish, a top coat and an orange stick.

Without using any water, file your friend's nails and gently push back the cuticles using the orange stick. This is important because any skin that sticks to the nail bed will make the polish lift up, making it easy to peel off. Next, rub the nail cleanser over all the nails using a lint-free wipe. Some kits have them but if not, you can get them at beauty supply stores for about $5 a pack. It's important to use this instead of cotton balls because cotton leaves tiny fibers that can mess up a manicure.

Next, apply the base color in a thin layer, then dry or cure it using the LED or UV lamp for about 30 to 60 seconds. Curing time will depend on the kit's instructions, so follow them carefully because under or over curing the gel can lead to chips and smudges. Next, apply the first coat of colored polish, then cure before applying the second coat, and cure again. Finally, paint on a thin layer of topcoat and place the hand under the lamp for the final curing.

After this, nails might feel a bit sticky, but this is normal. Simply saturate another lint-free wipe with the nail cleanser, and go over all ten nails. Now, your loved one has dry and super-shiny nails that stay that way for at least 2 weeks.

Chapter 9 - Hand Care and Manicure Maintenance

As with any gift, your loved one may want to preserve the beauty and neatness of the manicure which you so lovingly gave them. Though everyday life can lead to the inevitable chipping of nail polish and broken nails, there are ways for them to prolong the life of a manicure.

Before they leave your place, you can give them a small tube of hand cream, a small bottle of nail polish, or a stress ball as a token. These gifts will remind them to take care of their hands and nails until it's time for the next manicure. As you give them the manicure, you can dispel small bits of info or advice that will surely help them maintain the beauty and well-being of their hands.

First, advise your loved ones to regularly perform self-massage on their hands twice a day, usually after performing chores or after hours spent in front of a computer, and again before bedtime. The hand cream which you gave them can be used for this. Ask them to work the cream into the cuticles as well to moisturize them.

For stiff and aching hands, tell your friends to refrain from cracking their knuckles as this can lead to damaged joints. Instead, they can use a stress ball to relieve any stiffness in the hands.

Should they happen to chip their manicure, a simple solution is to buff the chip to smoothen the nail surface, then paint a similar shade on the chip in two thin coats. Next, apply a topcoat to seal it and restore shine.

To keep the manicure looking good, have your loved ones apply topcoat every 3 days because polish tends to gets dull after using harsh soaps and cleansers which are commonly found at home.
To maintain a gel manicure, regular moisturizing of the nails is the key to help nails look good. If your friend does not like the feel of hand cream, recommend a cuticle oil in a handy pen form. Good brands to try are Sally Hansen Maximum Growth Cuticle Pen, The Body Shop Almond Nail and Cuticle Oil, and Avon Nail Experts Cuticle Oil Pen.

To protect the hands and nails, have them apply sunscreen on the backs of the hands, as these are often overlooked when applying sunscreen. If a hand cream contains some SPF, that's even better since it eliminates the need to buy multiple products. Lotions and creams such as Molton Brown Soothing Hand Lotion SPF 15 and The Body Shop Wild Rose Hand Cream SPF 15 will help protect the hands from the harsh rays of the sun which causes skin cancer and premature wrinkling.

Our hands do a lot of work and are subject to stress and exposure to the elements every day, so it's important to care for them. By giving a manicure, your family and friends are pampered and cared for, and you have lavished them with attention which sometimes, is sorely needed by the busiest and most neglected of family members and friends. Take the time to do one today for someone who you think needs it the most. And, don't forget to give yourself one too. Everyone needs a little tender loving care once in a while.

Chapter 10-Benefits of Getting a Pedicure

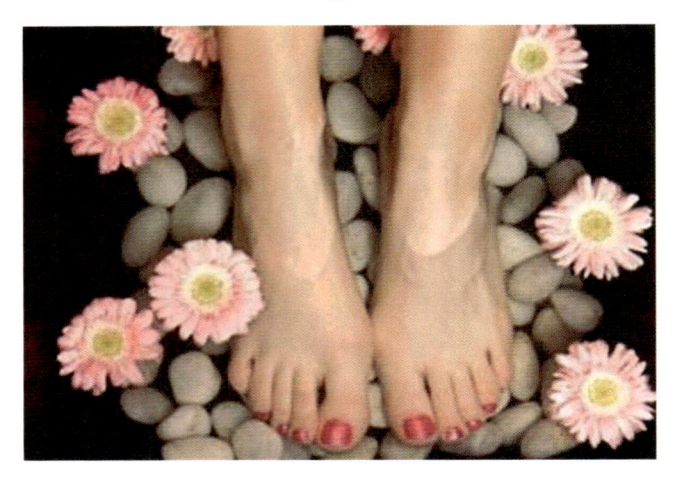

Staying healthy and well-groomed is an important aspect of everyday living. Aside from preventing disease and infection, being clean and groomed can contribute to the overall well-being of anyone. A person who is well-turned out seems to stand a little straighter, smile a little more, and has more confidence than someone who has been neglectful of his or her appearance.

Nowadays, establishments where one can get groomed seem to pop up on every corner. Of course, not everyone has the time and resources to go and visit a spa or a salon. If you have a friend or family member who you think is in sore need of pampering, giving them a pedicure in the comforts of your own home can be a very welcome treat.

Why a pedicure? Aside from having shiny, pretty toenails, there are health benefits to be gained from getting a pedicure. Cutting and shaping the toenails prevents them from growing inwards, more commonly known as ingrown nails. Also, removing dirt from under the toenails can prevent disease and bad bacteria from spreading. Unpleasant foot odors can also be remedied by a well-executed pedicure.

Slipping the feet into a warm basin of water with essential oils has health benefits. Depending on the type of oil being used, it can soothe, refresh, relax or calm the senses.

Exfoliating the feet can help prevent corns and bunions, which can be painful and hard to remove. Calluses can also be sloughed away, eliminating uneven pressure on feet. Plus, cell turnover is encouraged, revealing softer and smoother skin.

Massage is also part of the pedicure process, and this can help ease aches and pains. A person's legs and feet are subjected to constant impact and pressure, considering that the average person takes about 8000 to 10,000 steps daily. A quick massage is enough to soothe and reduce stress. It can also stimulate blood circulation which helps improve the appearance of the skin. People of all ages will surely benefit from a soothing massage done at least twice a month.

Apart from all these reasons, the simple act of giving a pedicure can be a thoughtful gesture to those who need it the most. Cutting toenails can be an ordeal for some people who cannot bend far enough to reach their feet. It can be quite a contortionist act for some, and it can also be daunting for those people who don't know how to care for their own toenails. Moreover, giving a pedicure is also a form of touch therapy. People who would need this the most are those who feel harassed and stressed by everyday life, or those who suffer from loneliness and depression. The time spent grooming a loved one's feet might only be a pedicure for some, but to the recipient, it is a sign of caring.

And the most obvious benefit from a pedicure is the sight of clean, polished toenails, just in time for the summer when people reach for sandals or flip flops instead of more concealing footwear. Often, the simple sight of well-groomed hands and feet can be enough to boost self-esteem and confidence.

Chapter 11 - Who Should and Shouldn't Get a Pedicure?

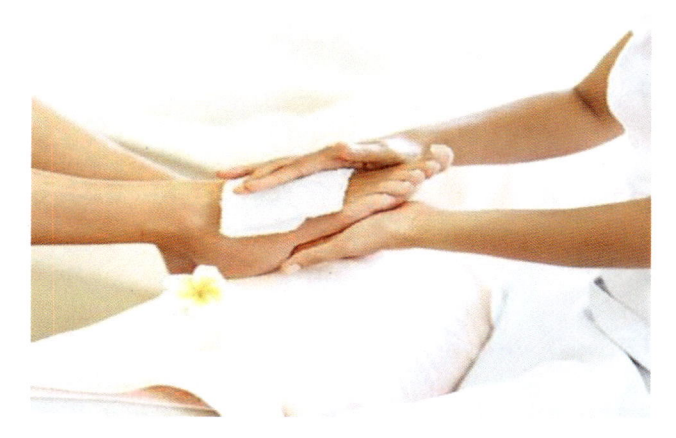

Giving a friend or a relative a pedicure is one way to pamper and care for them. However, there are some people with certain ailments or who are undergoing treatments that are advised not to get pedicures.

For instance, people with diabetes would do well not to get pedicures because they are prone to foot infections. One small nick while trimming the toenails can cause a life threatening infection. Because of this, only medically supervised technicians may perform a pedicure on a diabetic.

Likewise, anyone who is undergoing chemotherapy or immune suppression for a bone or cell stem transplant should not get a pedicure unless they have permission from their doctor.
So who should get a pedicure?

Look to the ones who seem to need the pampering the most. Got a pregnant friend? She is probably in need of some help when it comes to caring for her feet since her growing stomach can make it difficult to reach for her toes. Spending some time massaging her legs and feet will be a soothing and relaxing experience for her, since pregnancy comes with its share of different aches and pains.

An elderly relative in need of some attention will also appreciate the gesture. A lot of older people suffer from touch deprivation, especially those who are institutionalized. The need for physical closeness with another human being stays with us throughout our lives, and those who are older and left in the care of nurses or caretakers lack the attention, care and loving touch that only a relative can give.

Men may also appreciate a pedicure, though they may initially grumble about it being a girly activity. No man has ever complained about having neatly trimmed toenails, and few ever say no to the massage that accompanies a pedicure treatment. This may also be the perfect time to teach them about buffing, which makes the nails shiny sans clear polish.

Got a friend or family member who seems to have no time or money to spare for a professional pedicure? Offer them a 30-minute pedicure on a weekend, for free. Most salons or manicure places charge about $15 and up for the service, so a person who's on a tight budget will surely want a pedicure, free of charge.

Kids can also be part of the fun as pedicures involve a lot of fun aspects such as the foot bath and polishing. Watch a little girl's face light up as you paint their toenails with some glittery pink polish. Or paint their nails with all the colors of the rainbow. With a child, you can be creative when it comes to the choice and design of toenail polish.

Basically, anyone who needs a little pampering and attention will surely appreciate a pedicure. It is a gesture that is thoughtful and caring, and only takes a little time and effort to do. So set aside a weekend and make a treat of it. All the recipients will surely be grateful, and who knows, you could get one in return too.

How to Give a Home
Manicure & Pedicure

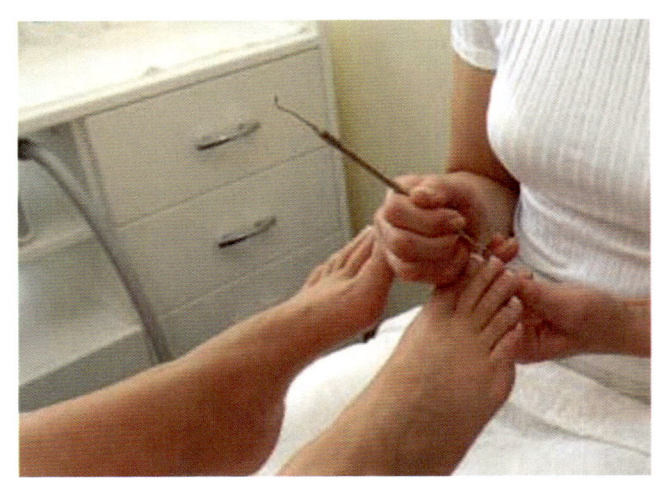

Chapter 12 - Setting the Stage for a Pedicure Party

A one-on-one pedicure is enjoyable, but a pedicure party is even more so. Pedicure parties can be a great way to have lots of fun, especially when shared with family and friends. It's a relaxing and enjoyable way to bond and share stories, and everyone leaves with groomed and freshly painted toenails. To have a good time, some planning may be in order before the day of the party.

- **Make a guest list**. If you are the only one who is going to perform the pedicures, plan on inviting 2 to 3 family members or friends to the party. Consider inviting people who already know each other to keep the conversations flowing. If you want to go all out, print some invitations and give them to each recipient. Or simply send them an e-vite or text message. At this point you should plan on giving your guests at least 30 minutes each for a pedicure, so 2 to 3 guests is really the ideal number unless there's another person to do the pedicures aside from you, then by all means invite more people.

- **Prepare the party venue.** The right place to have the party is some part of your home that will encourage relaxation, so your guests should be free to lounge around. The living room is the best option. Or, if you want to contain the spills and messes, you can have the party at your patio or sun room if you have one. It also helps if the area is well-lit so you can clearly see what you're doing once you start the pedicures. Provide plush seating and plenty of pillows for extra comfort. You should also have a low chair or ottoman where you can comfortably sit while you're doing the pedicure. Have the latest issues of fashion magazines on hand, and set up the TV and DVD player so that your guests can watch something while they're waiting for their turn. Depending on your guests and what they're in the mood for, some DVDs that you should have are classics such as Breakfast at Tiffany's or My Fair Lady; or iconic films of a particular decade such as The Breakfast Club (the 80's) or Clueless (the 90's). Have a few episodes of popular series available as well, such as Revenge or Downton Abbey. Or go completely girly and pop in Legally Blonde or Mean Girls. The choices are endless!

- **Have a few snacks for your guests.** Preferably, something that does not require a spoon and fork to eat it with. Appetizers and finger sandwiches are light yet will keep the hunger pangs away. Prepare a mix of savory and sweet treats such as mini tuna sandwiches, potato chips and some non-drippy dip, brownies and cookies. Have a selection of drinks to choose from such as fruit juice, coffee or tea. To evoke a spa-like vibe, serve cucumber sandwiches or grilled low fat mozzarella cheese sandwiches with tomatoes and basil that are cut into triangles, plus some healthful treats such as nuts and dried fruit, and set pitchers of lemon water for guests to help themselves. It's also good to tailor-fit your menu for your guests. A kiddie spa party will call for chips, oatmeal or chocolate cookies- just make sure not to overdo the sugar. If your guests are men, serve heartier fare such as grilled sandwiches with non-messy filling. The thing to remember is to serve nothing fussy, messy, greasy or anything that will fall apart at the first bite, such as tacos. It might not be a good idea to serve alcoholic drinks at a pedicure party, so stick to non-alcoholic beverages. Have your guests eat before the actual pedicure.

- **Prepare individual tools for your guests.** Each one should have their own emery board, orange wood sticks and towels when you do the pedicures. Don't use just one tool or implement for everybody. You can find all the things you need from the dollar store or from any supermarket. Have the same number of plastic basins as the number of guests you have. These basins will be used for the foot bath. Display at least 4 types of essential oils, at least 10 colors of nail polish to choose from, and a few towels on hand. Providing each guest with inexpensive rubber flip flops will also be a thoughtful gesture as this type of footwear ensures that carefully-painted nail polish will not be smudged and ruined.

- **At the end of the party, hand out some party favors for your guests.** The flip flops which you've provided earlier can serve as party favors. Get some inexpensive, colorful pairs in the right size. Another cute idea is to send your guests home with a bottle of new nail polish so they can touch up the pedicure once it chips.

With a little time and organization, your pedicure party will surely be a memorable event for all.

How to Give a Home
Manicure & Pedicure

Chapter 13 - Items You'll Need to Prepare for a Pedicure

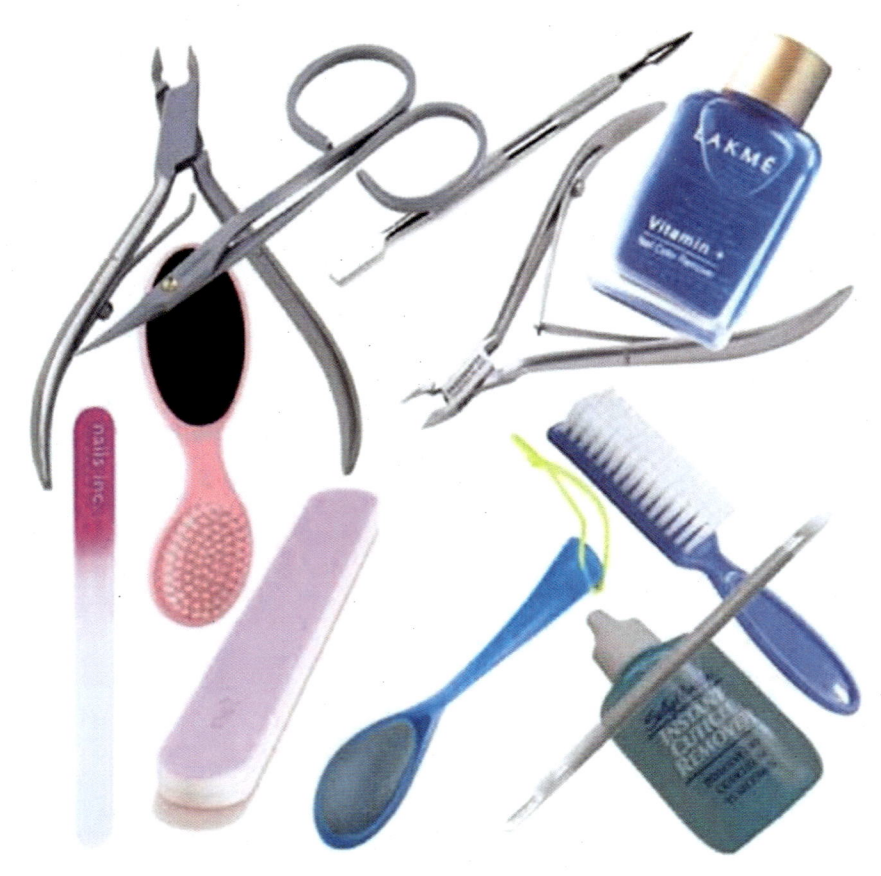

Before inviting a loved one or a friend to come over for a pedicure, it is necessary to have the right tools on hand to be able to perform a professional-grade pedicure. It's not enough to just swipe on nail polish and call it a day. There are several steps to follow- soaking, trimming, shaping, cleansing, massaging, and polishing, and each step comes with its own set of materials. Here is a list of things that you need to prepare:

- **A plastic basin,** big enough for both feet. Though the pedicure vibrating baths sold in beauty supply stores are great, you don't have to invest in them. A simple basin can hold enough soapy water for a relaxing foot soak.
- **Essential oils.** A few drops added to the foot soak can be soothing and can be a source of aromatherapy. Peppermint or mint oil invigorates and freshens and lavender oil has a calming effect. If you have blended oils you can also use those. Or, forego the oils and make milk soaks to soften and heal dry skin. You can use a cup of whole milk and add that to warm water, or buy specially formulated milk soaks from the drug store or beauty supply store.
-
- **Nail trimmer.** There are ones that are specially made to clip toenails. They're usually bigger than the average nail clipper, ideal for cutting tough toe nails.
- **Emery boards.** After clipping the nails, use this to file nails into the desired shape. You can get several at a very low price.
- **Orange sticks.** These are used to gently push back the cuticles and remove dirt underneath the nails.
- **Nail brush.** For scrubbing away dirt from the surface of the nails.
- **Foot file.** For exfoliating the soles of the feet. Good for sloughing away dry skin and calluses.
- **Nail polish remover.** If possible, get some that are acetone-free. Acetone-based removers are drying and can damage the nail.
- **Foot lotion or body lotion.** This will be used during the massage. Specially formulated lotions or moisturizers for the feet have anti-bacterial properties and often contain mint for a cooling effect. Or you can use regular body lotion.

- **Cotton balls.** For removing old nail polish and for cleaning up any smudges or any stray polish on the cuticles.
- **Nail buffer.** It gives the nails a glossy appearance, so it's perfect for anyone who doesn't like to use nail polish. It's about 3 times the size of a regular emery board, and it has 3 to 4 multi-colored surfaces.
- **Nail polish.** Prepare a selection of at least 10 colors, ranging from nude, pale colors, pastels, bright colors, and darks. Start with the classic five colors- a clear polish, a cream-colored one, a beige-nude one, a light pink one, and a true red polish. Then add more if you choose to do so.
- **Extras.** Nail stickers, a top coat and a base coat of nail polish and cuticle cream are all nice to have, but these are optional items.
- **Towels.** Have several medium-sized towels on hand.

You can purchase all these things at a drugstore or beauty supply store. Also, check the dollar store for cute and practical finds.

Chapter 14 - The First Step- A Foot Soak

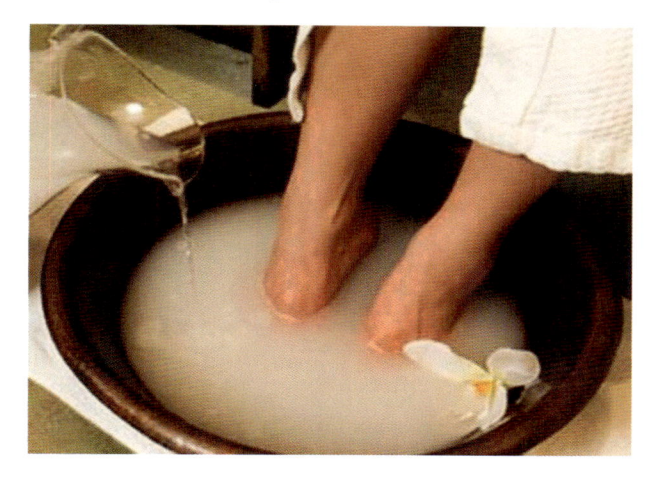

Before you grab that bottle of nail polish, some things have to be done first to be able to give a good pedicure. In salons, they usually have you soak your feet in a bubbling pedicure tub first. At home, you can do the same with a basin of warm water, some moisturizing liquid soap, and a couple of drops of essential oil.

Why should you let your friend or family member have a foot soak first? This step is important because it cleanses and disinfects the feet, softens the toenails which makes it easier to trim, and softens the cuticles, making it easier to push back for a neat look.

How should you prepare a foot soak? First, get a plastic basin big enough to put both feet in. Next, pour some warm water in to the basin, making sure that it's neither too hot nor too cool. Then, pour in a few drops of any liquid soap and mix it with the water to create a bubbly, light foam.

Now, add a few drops of essential oil to the foot bath. You should have a few different types on hand for your friend or relative to choose from. Remember to put in only a few drops because these oils are highly concentrated. Various oils have different aromatherapy benefits, and here are the top choices of essential oils used in professional nail salons:

- Peppermint- this is one of the most familiar oils and is commonly used in nail salons. It has a fresh scent and can help you stay alert and awake. It's also good for someone who's suffering from a slight headache or a clogged nose.
- Lavender- this oil has anti-bacterial properties and promotes a calming and relaxing effect. It also has healing properties and is especially effective in treating minor scrapes, cuts or burns. It can be used to treat athlete's foot. If your loved one is in need of stress relief and relaxation, this oil is recommended to be added into the foot soak.
- Tea tree oil- this has medicinal and healing properties, and those suffering from athlete's foot, itching, corns and sinusitis will greatly benefit from this oil.
- Rose oil- this is good for stress relief and can be very comforting. It's also good for those with mature skin.
- Orange oil- this oil is a big favorite. It's versatile and has a very uplifting effect, so if your loved one is in need of some cheer, a few drops of orange oil in the foot soak will help.

Let your loved one soak their feet for about 5 minutes. You can also do a light scrub on the feet and lower legs if you want, using a foot scrub or a mixture of olive oil and sugar. Avoid salt scrubs because they can irritate and can cause tiny scratches.

After soaking, rinse with more warm water and pat legs and feet dry with a soft towel.

Chapter 15 - Cutting and Shaping the Toenails

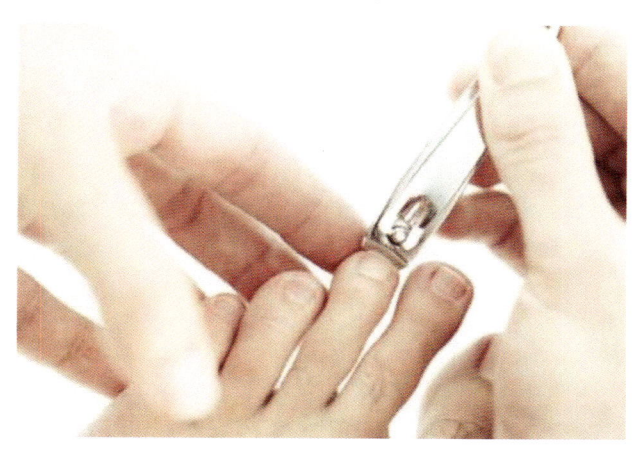

One of the most vital things to do when giving a pedicure is cutting and shaping the toenails. This has to be done carefully, paying attention to keeping every nail within the same length and shape.

Longer toenails used to be a big hit during the 80's, but now, more women are opting to have shorter nails. Aside from being more hygienic, it's also more practical. Long toenails are more prone to breakage, splitting, and infection- so keep them short.

Ideally, cutting the nails should be immediately done after the foot soak. Toenails are still soft from the soak, so that makes it easier to cut. Using toenail clippers (which are bigger than typical fingernail clippers), start trimming the nail from one side, going to the other side. Never snip the nail at the middle because this can cause the nail to split. Take care not to cut off too much because this can be painful. Ideally, the length of the nail should be just at the tip or slightly extend the tip of the toe.

After clipping the toenails, filing them should be the next step. Use an emery board for this purpose. There are many kinds available in the market, and some prefer to use a steel file, but if you're new to giving pedicures it's best to start with an emery board. File each nail from side to side, using short, quick strokes. Avoid filing the fingertips because the surface of an emery board is abrasive to the skin.

Now it's time to push back the cuticles. Apply a little bit of cuticle remover if you have it. This doesn't actually remove the cuticles like it says on the label, but it makes them soft enough to push back. Never attempt to push back dry cuticles because they are more prone to tearing. Next, get an orange stick and gently push back the cuticles while they're still moist. Then, carefully run the tip of the stick along the base of the nail to remove excess cuticle or any dead skin.

Some nail technicians cut the cuticles to make them look neater. It is advisable not to do this because the cuticle protects the root of the nail from infection. So just push them back gently, and never ever attempt to remove the cuticles in any way.

If you're a novice at giving pedicures, all the steps that have been indicated in this chapter should be done carefully. Also, it would be wise to know the medical history of the pedicure's recipient before you do any of these steps. For instance, a diabetic relative should not get a pedicure unless done by a medically supervised technician because one small break in the skin can lead to a life threatening infection. If your loved one is diabetic, simply have them do the foot soak and file the nails to shorten them.
It is also advisable to assign an emery board and an orange stick for each loved one to lessen the risk of cross contamination during pedicures.

Chapter 16- Exfoliation

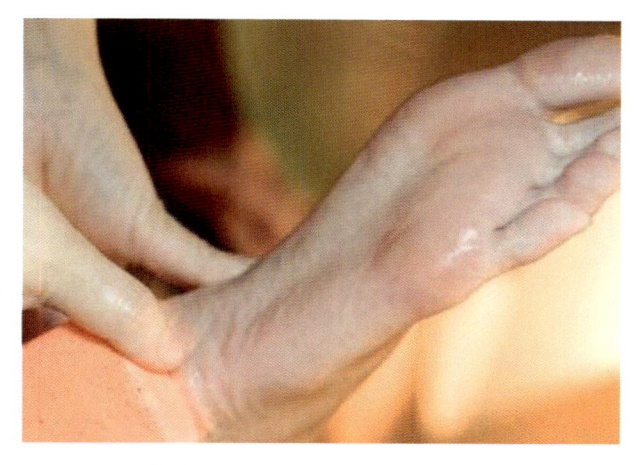

Exfoliation is one of the most beneficial things you can do to make the skin look great. The sloughing action removes dead skin, improves circulation, and reveals healthy, fresh skin. As we get older, regular exfoliation is a must because the shedding of old skin cells slows down over time. Look at a child's skin- it is positively glowing and radiant because skin cells are shed at a rapid pace. As adults, we need a little help to aid the cell renewal process to achieve the desired results.

During a pedicure, exfoliation is done to remove the dry and hard skin on the heels and soles of the feet brought about by walking and ill-fitting shoes. Women who regularly wear high heels will often have a myriad of foot problems such as corns, calluses, and dry and darkened heels. Exfoliation can help remedy these problems.

Exfoliation should be performed right after clipping and shaping the toenails. Here are the steps to follow:
- After cutting and filing the toenails, refill the basin with warm water and let your loved one soak their feet once more for 5 minutes.

- Have some scrubs and an exfoliating implement on hand. There are numerous scrubs available in the market, with the ones containing ground apricot proving to be particularly effective. For a more cost effective alternative, simply look to your pantry for ingredients for a DIY scrub. Mix a half cup of olive oil with 5 spoons of sugar. Stir the mixture well, and apply to feet and legs with an upwards scrubbing motion. Avoid salt scrubs as they can be highly irritating and can sting freshly shaved legs.

- Rinse the legs. For the feet, an exfoliating implement with a more abrasive surface is needed to tackle hardened skin and calluses. A pumice stone or foot file will work. Never use a metal foot file unless you're comfortable using it as this can injure the skin. Using the stone or foot file, go over the soles of the feet, paying particular attention to the balls of the feet and heels. After that, rinse, and pat the feet dry with a clean towel.

-

Immediately, you will notice a difference in the skin's appearance. No more dull, lackluster skin on the feet and legs, only smoother, softer and glowing skin.

You're almost close to completing the pedicure. The next chapters will discuss massage and polishing.

Chapter 17 – Massage

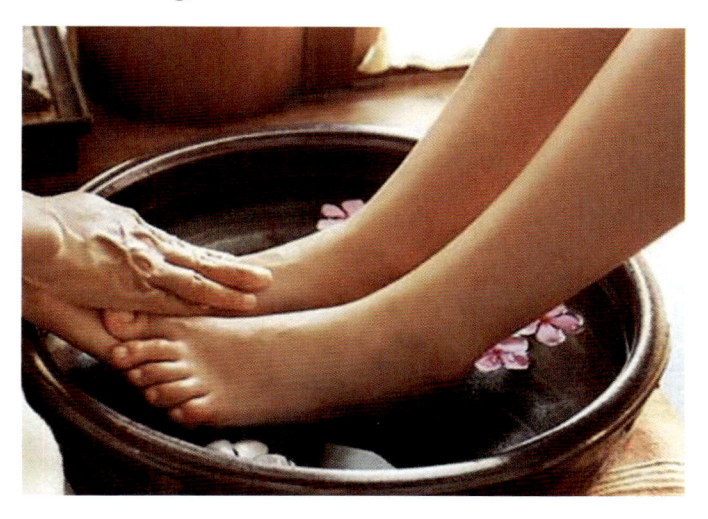

A foot massage is one of the most caring and thoughtful things that you can give a friend or family member. It does not cost anything and it will only take about 5 to 10 minutes to do. The recipient of a foot massage will experience relief from stress, have improved blood circulation, and any pains and foot ache will be remedied.

This part of the pedicure can also be a very nurturing and bonding experience for you and your loved one. So make this part count, and follow this guide to performing a wonderful foot and leg massage.
- The massage should be done after exfoliation and prior to applying nail polish. Make sure that the legs and feet of your loved one are completely dry before you start.
- You will need some massage oil or lotion to give your hands a little slip to make the massage more relaxing. Oils such as sweet almond oil is ideal because it is slow to be absorbed into the skin. You'll want to keep the surface of the skin moist while massaging, so formulas that are

thicker or richer are preferable than light lotions. Body creams or body butters work well too. If you don't have any of these, regular body lotion will do. Just apply more once the lotion gets absorbed.
- Ask your loved one to lean back and relax, and have an ottoman or cushioned chair ready for them to prop their feet up. Place a towel on the chair to protect it from oils or creams. Start the massage with the right foot.
- Using both thumbs, stroke the foot starting from the tops of the foot with an even pressure, and your thumbs should be stroking upwards and sliding back from you as you continue towards the heel. Repeat this step at least 4 times.
- Guide the foot to do ankle rotations. Hold the ankle, then with your other hand, grasp the top of the foot and slowly rotate doing 5 turns clockwise, then 5 turns counter clockwise.
- Next, do some toe pulls. Starting from the base of the toe, slowly pull the toe and slide your fingers upwards. Don't do a sudden, jerky pulling motion because this can dislocate the toes.
- Massage the arch of the foot by pushing the heel of your hand right at the arch, going upwards towards the toes.
- Massage the lower leg, using long, upward strokes with your hands. Remember to keep the pressure even. At this point you might need to apply more massage oil or lotion. Remember to always keep the skin moist to make it easier for you to do the massage.
- Do the same steps with the other foot.

If you are trained in reflexology, you may want to do a reflexology massage instead of a regular massage. Studies have shown that when certain parts of the feet are massaged or if you apply steady pressure to these parts, they can relieve minor ailments such as stuffy nose, headaches, stomach ache and lower back ache.

While performing the massage, it is important that you stay relaxed and in a positive mood. Remember that as you massage one person, energy flows from you to your loved one. So keep the good vibe going by taking your time, and just enjoy bonding with them.

How to Give a Home
Manicure & Pedicure

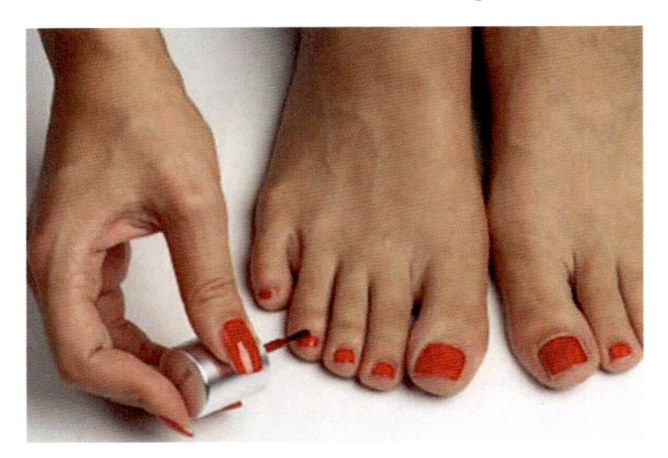

Chapter 18 - The Final Touches- Buffing and Polishing

We're now at the final and most important part of the pedicure- buffing and polishing the toenails. This last step is what people look forward to, since this makes the toenails look good and shiny. Proper technique and the right products will surely make a difference when it comes to this step.

If the recipient of the pedicure is a man or if someone does not like nail polish, you can buff the nails instead. Buffing makes the surface of the nail smooth and gives it a shiny, glassy finish. Some celebrities such as Sarah Jessica Parker and Howard Stern have even been spotted while having their nails buffed at swanky nail salons. It just goes to show that this is a good way to finish off a pedicure if your loved one prefers to have unpolished toenails.

Nail buffers come in all kinds of sizes and colors, but to get the most professional results, get a 3-sided nail buffer. This is shaped like an emery board, is thrice as large as one and is pliable. It has different colored surfaces and the texture of each surface varies from gritty to smooth, and they're usually numbered to help you know which side to use first.

To buff the toenails, start with the side with the number 1 and go over the surface of the nail with it. This removes any deep seated dirt and files down any bumps on the nail. Follow with the side with the number 2 on it. This eliminates ridges on the nails. Finish with the number 3 side, and buff the nails with a quick side to side motion to get a glassy finish. You can give your loved ones their very own buffer for them to maintain the shiny appearance of their toenails at home.

If buffing sounds easy enough, putting on nail polish might be trickier than expected. Aside from the smudges and uneven globs and drips, it can be quite trying to really get it done right. But with the right products and technique, nail polish application will soon become a cinch.

Have these things ready: toe separators, cotton, orange wood stick, nail polish remover, nail polish, top coat- this is the clear, final layer that goes on top of the colored nail polish.
You should have several colors of nail polish to choose from. If you have no idea what your loved one might prefer, have some of the classics and tried and true colors on hand. These colors are:
- Clear- no hint of color at all, and gives a shiny finish. This can be used in place of a top coat.
- Cream- ivory white or a golden cream is ideal for doing a clean wash of pale color or for French pedicures.
- Nude beige- gives a clean and classy finish to toes, perfect for a wide range of skin tones.
- Pale pink- for a feminine hint of color
- True red- incredibly flattering on toes.

Aside from these 5 shades, you can incorporate other fun colors such as corals or purples, and why not throw in a sparkly polish in the mix too?

How to Give a Home
Manicure & Pedicure

To start, let your loved one wear a toe separator. Then, wipe away any residue on the nails with a clean towel. Start by painting in 3 strokes, one in the middle, then on either side of the nail. Make sure to apply a thin coat of polish to prevent globs. Apply a second coat of nail polish using the 3 stroke method. Then, top it off with a layer of top coat or clear polish. To clean up any mistakes or smudges beyond the nail bed, wrap a bit of cotton around the pointy end of an orange stick. Dip it in polish remover, then use it to clean up stray polish around the cuticles. It takes about 15 to 20 minutes for nail polish to dry, so have your loved one relax while the nail polish dries.

And you're done- a perfectly executed pedicure, lovingly performed by you.

With time, preparation, and the willingness to care and pamper family and friends, anyone can do a good pedicure. It's a worthwhile activity to show your love for the people who matter the most.

Printed in Great Britain
by Amazon.co.uk, Ltd.,
Marston Gate.